30 Best Smoothies for Instant Weight loss: *Blend your way to a better you, your journey to a healthier and happier you.*

Gifted E. Davids

Copyright

NOTEPAD

INTRODUCTION

You must be committed to losing weight if you are reading this right now.

Even though this seems straightforward and commonplace, I would nonetheless Say it! Soft drink consumption is unhealthy! really detrimental!

The preferred beverage for millions of people around the globe is soft drinks.

It is common knowledge that carbonated beverages are unhealthy, although despite this information, some people continue to do business with them, most likely because it is simply affordable and accessible.

It is important to understand that sugar-filled beverages raise the risk of obesity, type 2 diabetes, and fat storage in the body, cardiac problems, and further long-term ailments.

Just pointing out a problem or a solution is insufficient, they (solutions) must be made available. This led to the creation of smoothies.

WHAT ARE SMOOTHIES?

Smoothies are thick drinks created by blending raw fruits or veggies combined with additional seasonings to taste by the individual. Smoothies, as opposed to fruit drinks, need the blending of entire
fruits without additional additives such as preservatives additives, so all of its nutritional value is present.

It's also crucial to remember that smoothies include fruit fiber, which aids in digestion and increases its nourishment level.

Some also incorporate herbs and spices, such as ginger, for higher nutritious content.

If your goal to reduce weight is sincere and committed, Prepare to give up soft drinks and embrace Smoothies, instead!

Furthermore, In the ever-evolving world of health and wellness, the quest for effective and sustainable weight loss solutions remains a top priority for many individuals. While there is no magic pill to shed excess pounds overnight, a well-balanced diet and regular exercise are crucial components of any weight loss journey. However, for those looking to add a tasty twist to their efforts, smoothies can be a delicious and nutritious addition to their arsenal.

Smoothies offer a convenient and enjoyable way to incorporate a variety of nutrients into your daily routine. When crafted thoughtfully, these blended beverages can be not only satisfying and flavorful but also supportive of your weight loss goals.

In this guide, we'll introduce you to the 30 best smoothies for instant weight loss, each carefully designed to help you on your journey to a healthier and happier you!

Here are our 30 Best smoothies and their benefits we are going to be talking about, that will give you to your dream body:

1.Green Powerhouse Smoothie:
Packed with leafy greens like spinach and kale, this vibrant green smoothie is a nutrient-rich powerhouse that can kickstart your weight loss journey.

2. Berry Blast Smoothie:
Antioxidant-rich berries, such as strawberries, blueberries, and raspberries, come together in this sweet and tangy blend to support metabolism and fight cravings.

3. Tropical Paradise Smoothie:
Escape to the tropics with a smoothie that combines the goodness of pineapple, coconut,

and mango to boost your metabolism and promote satiety.

4. Protein-Packed Peanut Butter Banana Smoothie:

A delicious combination of protein-packed peanut butter, bananas, and Greek yogurt provides a creamy and satisfying option for curbing hunger and building lean muscle.

5. Detox Green Smoothie: This detoxifying blend features ingredients like cucumber, mint, and lemon to aid in digestion and promote a healthy gut.

6. Avocado-Kale Smoothie: Rich in healthy fats and fiber, the avocado-kale smoothie can keep you feeling full and energized, making it easier to resist unhealthy snacks.

7. Chia Seed Delight: Chia seeds are known for their ability to absorb liquid and expand in the stomach, providing a feeling of fullness that can help curb overeating.

8. Oatmeal Breakfast Smoothie: Start your day with a wholesome oatmeal smoothie that combines oats, almond milk, and your favorite fruits for sustained energy and fewer cravings.

9. Spicy Mango-Carrot Smoothie: The inclusion of metabolism-boosting spices and the beta-carotene-packed carrot makes this smoothie a fiery yet effective choice for weight loss.

10. Cinnamon Apple Pie Smoothie: This guilt-free indulgence combines the flavors of apple pie with cinnamon to keep you feeling satisfied without the added sugar and calories.

11. Watermelon Cooler: Stay hydrated and curb your appetite with a refreshing watermelon smoothie that's perfect for hot summer days.

12. Ginger Turmeric Elixir: Ginger and turmeric are known for their anti-inflammatory properties, making this smoothie a potent choice for overall health and weight management.

13. Beet-Blueberry Beauty Blend: Beets are a superfood packed with vitamins and minerals, and when combined with blueberries, they create a delightful blend that supports your overall well-being.

14. Minty Fresh Smoothie: Mint not only adds a refreshing kick to your smoothie but can also help with digestion and reduce cravings.

15. Peachy Green Smoothie: The natural sweetness of peaches and the nutritional boost from spinach make this smoothie a tasty choice for weight loss.

16. Pumpkin Spice Delight: Savor the flavors of autumn year-round with this pumpkin spice smoothie that offers a healthier alternative to the seasonal favorite.

17. Chocolate Almond Dream: Indulge your sweet tooth with a chocolate almond smoothie that incorporates cocoa powder, almond milk, and a hint of sweetness without the guilt.

18. Spinach and Berry Protein Punch: This protein-rich smoothie is perfect for those looking to build muscle and support their weight loss goals.

19. Cranberries cleansers: These are known for their detoxifying properties, making this smoothie a perfect choice for a cleanse.

20. Aloe Vera Digestive Detox: Aloe vera can soothe the digestive system and assist in healthy weight management, making it a unique and refreshing addition to your weight loss journey.

21. Lemon-Ginger Zest Smoothie: This zesty blend features lemon and ginger to aid digestion and rev up your metabolism.

22. Blue-Green Algae Elixir: Spirulina and chlorella, two nutrient-dense blue-green algae, make this smoothie a powerful detoxifier and energy booster.

23. Pomegranate Passion Smoothie: Pomegranate seeds are rich in antioxidants and can help control your appetite and cravings.

24. Pineapple-Mint Slim Down: Pineapple's natural enzymes and mint's digestive properties come together to support healthy weight management.

25. Matcha Green Tea Zen: Matcha green tea is known for its metabolism-boosting qualities and can help increase fat oxidation.

26.Creamy Butternut Squash: This smoothie features butternut squash, which is low in calories and high in fiber, making it an ideal choice for weight loss.

27. Spinach-Strawberry Flax Fusion: Spinach, strawberries, and flax seeds combine to create a fiber-packed and delicious smoothie.

28. Cucumber-Celery Cool-Down: This hydrating smoothie is perfect for curbing cravings and keeping your body refreshed.

29. Moringa Magic: Moringa is a nutrient powerhouse, and this smoothie is an excellent way to incorporate it into your diet for weight loss.

30. Almond Joy Delight: Satisfy your sweet cravings with a healthier twist by blending almond milk, coconut, and a touch of cocoa for a guilt-free treat. And so on

As you embark on your weight loss journey, these 30 best smoothies can be your flavorful companions, providing you with essential nutrients, promoting satiety, and helping you reach your goals more effectively. Remember that while smoothies can play a valuable role in weight loss, it's important to maintain a balanced diet and exercise regularly for optimal results. Cheers to a healthier, happier, and more vibrant you

THE WEIGHT LOSS JOURNEY

1. GREEN POWERHOUSE SMOOTHIE

The name says it all: powerhouse. This smoothie is loaded with nutrients.

This one serving smoothie contains fiber, healthy fats, protein, and a variety of vitamins and minerals. I adore smoothies. What other dish contains spinach, microgreens, pear, kiwi, banana, hemp seeds, coconut oil, and honey? There are none that come to mind! Maybe a salad, but I don't always want to chew all that lettuce! Yaaak.

Not to mention the health benefits of this smoothie...Thank God for high-performance blenders.

Ingredients

- 1½ cups coconut milk or almond milk
- Extra large handful of organic spinach
- ¼ cup broccoli microgreens (or other leafy green of choice)
- 1 organic pear, cored
- 1 organic kiwi, peeled
- ½ banana
- 1 Tbsp. hemp seeds
- 1 Tbsp. coconut oil
- 1 tsp. raw honey

Instructions

Add all the ingredients in the order listed to a high-speed blender and blend on high until smooth

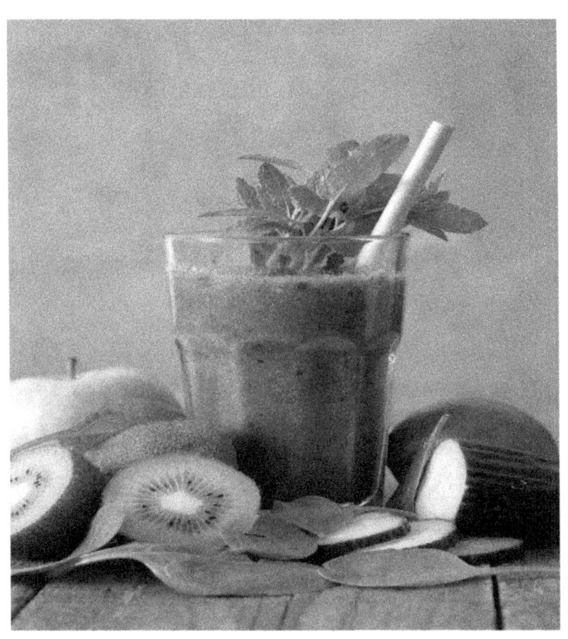

2. BERRY BLAST SMOOTHIE

These delicious and filling smoothies will definitely brighten up your summer! They're not only refreshing, but they're also simple to create. They'll be a big hit as a tasty summer treat!

Ingredients

- 3 cups mixed frozen berries raspberries, blueberries, blackberries, thawed slightly

- 1 cup fresh or frozen strawberries sliced (if using frozen thaw slightly first)
- 1 cup light vanilla yogurt
- 1 Tablespoon sugar
- 1 teaspoon vanilla extract
- 1 1/2 cups orange juice

Instructions

1. Add all of the ingredients inside a blender. Close with lid and blend until well combined. Pour into glasses and enjoy!
2. (If you like a thicker smoothie just use less juice.)

3.   TROPICAL   PARADISE SMOOTHIE

Ingredients

- ¼ cups apricot nectar or orange juice

- cup Cabot Low Fat Vanilla Bean Greek Yogurt
- 2 cups frozen mango chunks (about 9 ounces)

Directions

COMBINE juice, yogurt and mango in a blender; puree on high speed for about 45 seconds or until completely smooth.
SERVE immediately.

4.   PROTEIN-PACKED   PEANUT BUTTER BANANA SMOOTHIE

A simple and quick breakfast meal
While many people enjoy the ease of overnight oats, toast with jam, or a bowl of cold cereal for breakfast, I always feel hungry less than an hour

after eating a high carbohydrate breakfast with little protein.

Unlike many other quick breakfast options, this easy peanut butter banana smoothie recipe contains a good combination of protein, carbs, and healthy fats to keep you satisfied.

It can be really beneficial to have a nutritious breakfast drink in your time-saving recipe arsenal, especially on hurried Monday mornings.

Ingredients

- Banana
- Peanut butter
- Almond milk
- Greek yogurt
- Cinnamon

Direction

Add all ingredients in a blender,
Blend until smooth
Serve and enjoy.

5. DETOX GREEN SMOOTHIE

This Detox Smoothie tastes like a liquid vitamin! The components in this smoothie have been carefully selected to provide your body with nutrients without the use of any specialty powders or pricey supplements. Instead, you only need a few fruits and vegetables from your refrigerator!

- 1/2 cup water (or orange juice)
- 1 green apple
- 1/2 cup frozen pineapple chunks
- 1/2 frozen banana
- 1/2 inch fresh ginger , peeled and minced
- 1 cup fresh spinach
- small handful fresh cilantro
- 1 tablespoon fresh lime juice

INSTRUCTIONS

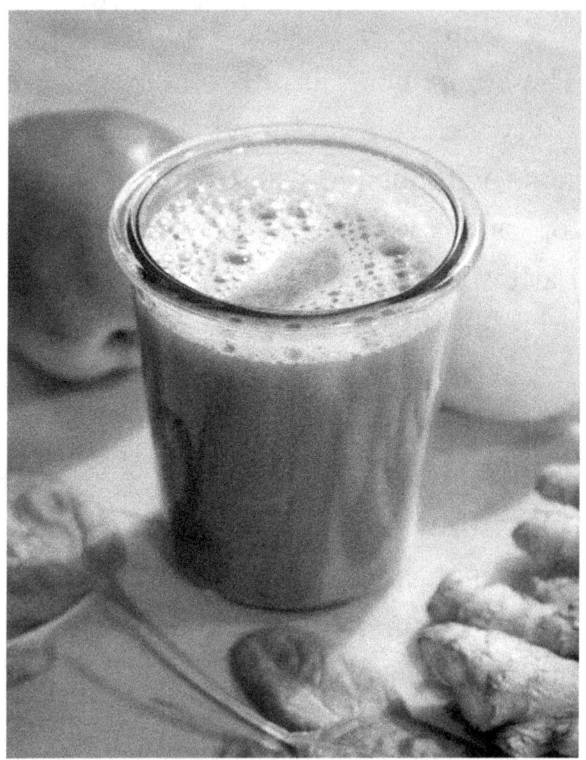

Combine all of the ingredients in a blender, and blend until smooth. Pour into a glass and serve right away.

If you don't have a high-speed blender, I recommend blending the spinach, cilantro, and ginger with the water first, to help break them down completely. Then add in the fruit and lime juice, and blend again.

6. AVOCADO - KALE SMOOTHIE

This creamy avocado smoothie comes together quickly, with only 5 ingredients, 1 blender, and 5 minutes. The base is made from frozen banana, which results in a creamy, naturally sweet base. The star ingredient is next: avocado! Avocado, which is high in fiber and healthful fats, makes this smoothie creamy, luscious, and thick, almost like a milkshake. Following that is dairy-free milk for a smooth and dreamy texture, followed by your favorite greens for fiber, nutrients, and a gorgeous green tint. The final component, protein powder, elevates this smoothie to the level of a meal.

7. CHIA SEEDS DELIGHT

INGREDIENTS

- ¼ cup organic raw chia seeds
- 1 ¾ cup homemade almond or hazelnut milk or, if not possible, a store-bought unsweetened brand
- 2 ½ teaspoon raw cacao powder
- ½ teaspoon vanilla extract
- 3 tablespoons coconut nectar
- Optional additional sweetener: stevia or xylitol

INSTRUCTIONS

In a bowl, combine the chia seeds.

In a blender, combine the almond milk, cacao powder, vanilla, coconut nectar, and stevia or xylitol until fully combined and the appropriate amount of sweetness is obtained. Mix in the chia seeds thoroughly.

Allow for at least 15 minutes before combining and serving.Enjoy!

8. OATMEAL BREAKFAST

Ingredients

- Berry and Oat Smoothie
- 1/2 cup rolled oats (125 ml)
- 1 cup milk dairy or non-dairy (250 ml)
- 1 Tbsp honey or agave (15 ml)
- 1/4 cup yogurt vanilla (60 ml)
- 1 cup berries strawberry, raspberry, blueberry or blackberry,
- 1 cup pineapple frozen, chunks (250 ml)
- 1 cup kale baby, packed (250 ml)
- 1 tbsp Peanut Butter and Banana Oat Smoothie
- 1 banana sliced and frozen, med-large

Apple Pie Oat Smoothie

- 1/2 cup rolled oats (125 ml)
- 1 cup milk dairy or non-dairy (250 ml)
- 1 Tbsp honey or agave (15 ml)
- 1/4 cup yogurt vanilla (60 ml)
- 6 applesauce cubes, frozen unsweetened
- 1/4 tsp cinnamon or apple pie spice (1 ml)

Instructions

Add all ingredients to a blender.

Cover tightly and pulse to chop fruit, then puree until smooth.

Taste and adjust sweetener, if necessary.

Serve immediately. (Note: smoothies will thicken on standing.)

9. SPICY MANGO-CARROT SMOOTHIE

Ingredients

- Carrots: Add 12 cups of ice or more to the blender to substitute fresh carrots and/or fresh mango (peeled and diced).
- A ripe mango, like an avocado or a peach, will give slightly when squeezed. When ripe, it should also smell fruity near the stem.

- Protein powder: 12 cup Greek yogurt or your preferred vanilla protein powder, Ginger to taste.

Step by step instructions

1. add orange juice, banana, mango, ginger and carrots in the blender

2. Blend until smooth and serve.

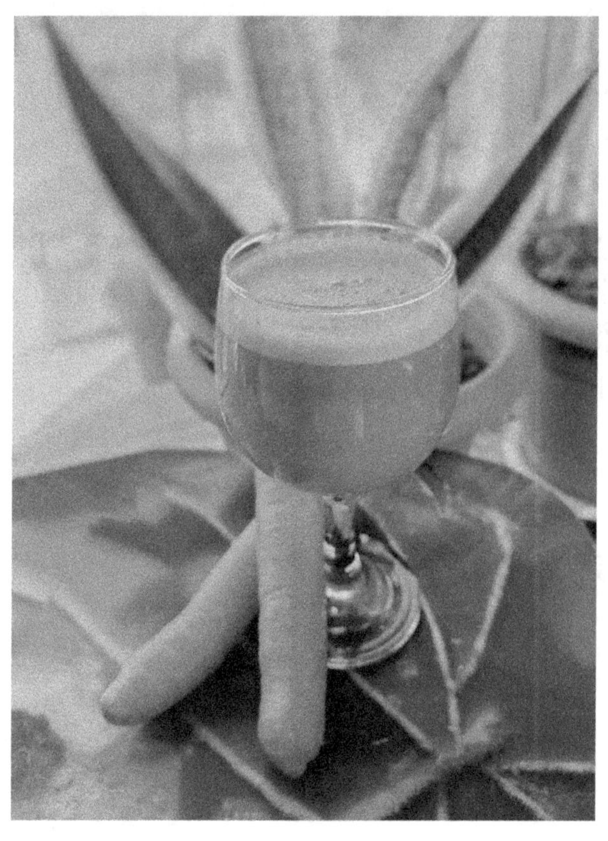

10.   CINNAMON   APPLE   PIE SMOOTHIE

Smoothie with Vegan Cinnamon Apple Pie
Simply include a frozen banana or two, a peeled apple, almond milk, almond butter, cinnamon, and nutmeg in a blender to make this vegan

cinnamon apple pie smoothie. Once combined, pour this apple-cinnamon smoothie into a glass and top with your favorite toppings. A few pinches of ground cinnamon and a sprinkle of shelled hemp seeds are my favorite additions.

- 1½ to 2 peeled, sliced, and frozen ripe and speckled bananas
- 1 peeled, seeded, and quartered apple
- 1 cup almond milk, vanilla
- 1 tbsp. almond butter
- 12 teaspoon cinnamon powder
- A pinch of freshly ground nutmeg
-

Topping Suggestions

The seeds of chia, walnuts ground cinnamon, apple slivers, and almonds spread.

Instructions

In a high-powered blender, combine the frozen bananas, apple, almond milk, almond butter, cinnamon, and nutmeg.

Blend for 1-2 minutes on high, or until smooth and creamy.

Pour into a glass, top with your favorite toppings, and serve.

11. WATERMELON COOLER

Nothing beats a refreshing drink on a hot summer day, which is why we're offering this recipe for a Refreshing Watermelon Cooler. This simple cocktail recipe offers a tasty combination of fresh watermelon and lemon juice. You'll be addicted after only one drink!

INSTRUCTIONS

In a large pitcher, combine watermelon puree, lemon juice, and sugar; mix until sugar is dissolved. Chill until ready to serve, or serve right away over ice..

Chill until ready to serve, or serve right away over ice.

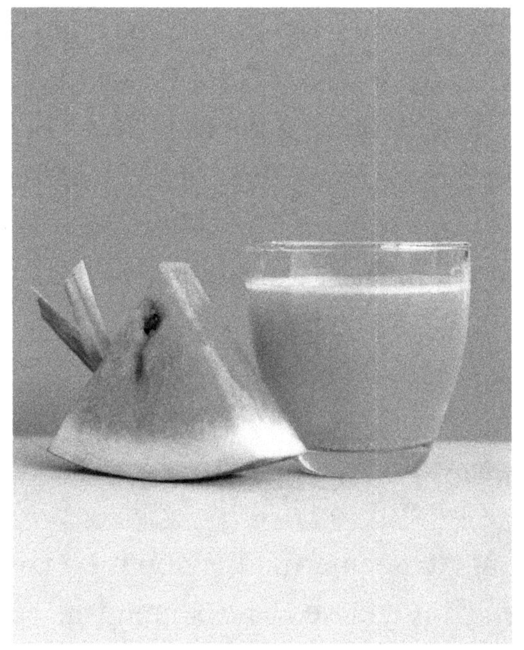

12. GINGER TURMERIC ELIXIR

In a juicer, combine the ginger, turmeric, oranges, and lemons. Once juiced, add water and pepper to taste. Fill your huge ice molds halfway with the freshly squeezed juice. Insert a basil leaf into each and gently toss. Freeze for at least 3 hours. When ready to use, take a frozen juice cube and cover it with boiling water. Allow your cube to melt before stirring! Feel free to add a dash of honey or your preferred sweetener. Drink chilled or warm for a warming elixir!

13. Beet-Blueberry Beauty Blend

This antioxidant-rich superfood smoothie will have you feeling invigorated and shining in no time. Anthocyanins, which are abundant in beets and blueberries, are potent antioxidants that minimize oxidative stress by neutralizing free radicals that can cause aging, sickness, and memory loss. Coconut oil contains lauric acid, which is a natural antibacterial, antifungal, and antiviral agent. It also improves energy expenditure rather than being stored as fat, which can contribute to more weight reduction in the long run. Because hemp seeds are high in fiber, protein, and healthy omega fats, this gorgeous, balanced smoothie is ideal for refueling after a workout!

Recipe:

- 1 juiced beet
- 1/2 cup fresh blueberries
- 1 cup nut or hemp milk
- 1 tablespoon of coconut oil
- 3 cubes of ice to taste, fresh honey

Combine all of the ingredients and serve!

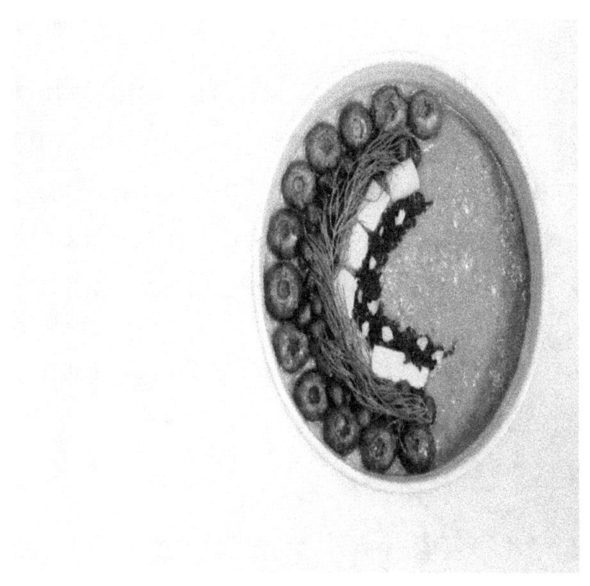

14. MINTY FRESH SMOOTHIE

Ingredients.

Frozen bananas make an excellent natural sweetener for smoothies like this Date Shake. They also contribute to the rich and creamy texture.

Spinach: Not only do spinach leaves add nourishment to this smoothie (hello, vitamins and iron), but they also contribute to its vibrant green hue.

Avocado: It contributes to the smoothie's green color and makes it super creamy. It's one of my favorite green smoothie ingredients (as shown in this Blueberry Banana Avocado Smoothie and this Cleansing Apple Avocado Smoothie).

Mint: Fresh mint leaves provide the essential cool, minty flavor. The leaves also contribute to the green color.

Almond Milk with Vanilla. For this recipe, I like to use vanilla almond milk as the liquid. The vanilla flavor complements the sweet and minty flavors perfectly.

Extract of peppermint. Adds a burst of minty flavor. Caution: a little goes a long way.

Sweetener. To add a touch of sweetness. Stevia, Truvia, honey, or maple syrup will all work nicely in this application.

15. PEACHY GREEN SMOOTHIE

INGREDIENTS

Two cups (480 ml) soy milk or any other type of milk

Two large (400 g), peeled and seeded apples

120 grams or 4 cups fresh spinach

480 grams, or 4 cups, frozen peach slices

Guidelines

After putting the ingredients in the Vitamix container according to the given order, cover it tightly.

Begin by using the blender at its lowest speed, then swiftly raise it to its maximum speed.

Blend for 30 to 45 seconds, or until desired consistency is achieved, pressing contents toward the blades with the tamper.

Chef's Remarks

Feel free to use any greens you have on hand or seasonal vegetables in place of the spinach. Consider making your own plant-based milk in your Vitamix.

16. PUMPKIN SPICE DELIGHT SMOOTHIE

An ideal breakfast for autumn!

Make a delicious, thick, and creamy pumpkin spice smoothie with ease using pumpkin puree. In addition to being high in fiber and carotenoids, such as beta-carotene, pumpkin is also a good source of vitamin A.

Add all ingredients in a blender.

- Almond milk, 12 ounces
- One banana
- one cup pureed pumpkin
- One mound Caramel
- One tablespoon of pure maple syrup, or as much as desired
- 1/4 tsp vanilla
- A tsp of cinnamon
- 8 tsp of nutmeg
- 1/8 teaspoon of clover
- Scoop of ice cubes

Serve and enjoy!!

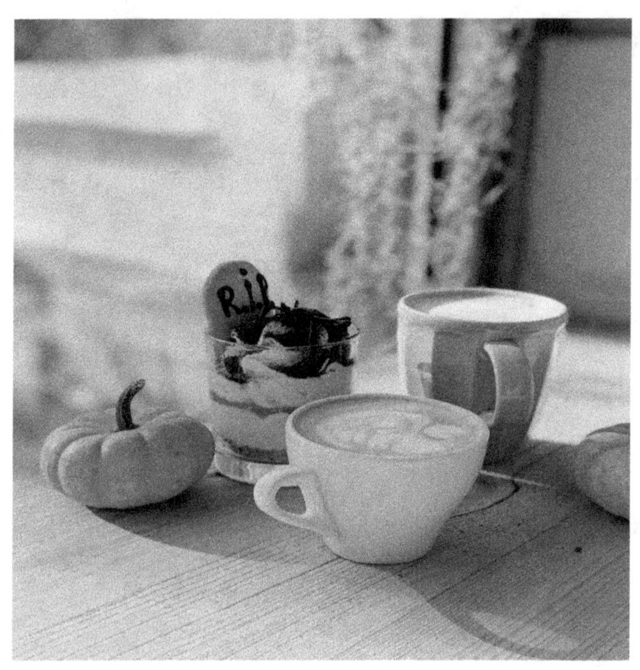

17. CHOCOLATE ALMOND DREAM

This specific smoothie is constructed with natural, simple ingredients, so you can definitely feel good about sipping it. Smoothies have to be very simple to make and made using items we usually have on hand in our household.

INGREDIENTS

Banana. Although I am aware that some people dislike bananas in smoothies, I don't think there is a better method to achieve an all-natural, sweet, and creamy texture. Furthermore, smoothies along with banana bread and muffins—are essentially our only chance of using up the enormous quantity of overripe bananas that we seem to be acquiring on a regular basis.

Nut milk. Although I like to use sweetened vanilla almond milk for this recipe, any kind will do. For a thinner smoothie, feel free to add an extra splash. To start, use 1/2 cup of milk for every frozen banana.

Cocoa mass. That chocolate has to come from someplace! For an added nutritional boost, you can also substitute protein powder with a chocolate taste.

Add-ins: cinnamon, chia seeds, etc. are optional. Add one or two teaspoons of your favorite addition for taste and nutrition. Oats or flax seeds also work nicely; for a creamier, richer texture, try adding a tablespoon of almond butter.

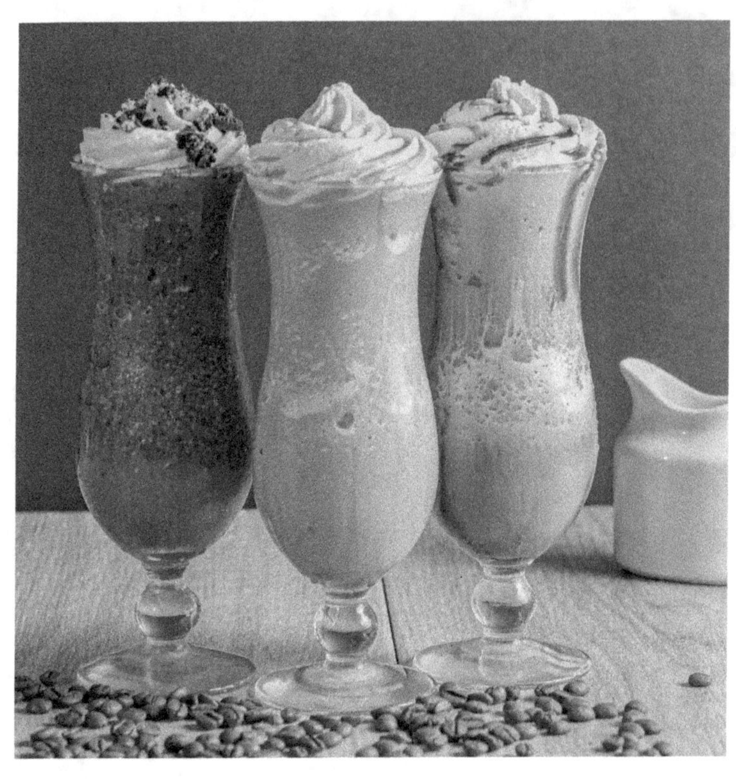

18. SPINACH AND BERRY PROTEIN PUNCH

We have jobs to prepare for, kids to feed, social media to monitor, and mornings are hectic times. My Berry Spinach Protein Smoothie is my go-to healthy breakfast recipe for folks who are busy and don't have a lot of time in the morning. I adore smoothies, don't get me wrong; I'm the resident smoothie expert here, but right now my kids and I are completely fascinated with this Berry Spinach Smoothie.

Components

Add your preferred combination of strawberries, blueberries, raspberries, or blackberries to any frozen or fresh berry dish. innately lively and pleasant.

Banana: Nutrient-dense, creamy, and sweet.

Greek yogurt: Provides extra creaminess and is packed with protein and good fats.

Protein powder: Boosts protein content and adds taste and sweetness.

Flaxseed meal: Rich in antioxidants, omega-3 fatty acids, and fiber, but largely tasteless.

Ginger: Provides vitamins and nutrients along with a crisp, vibrant flavor.

Cinnamon: A delectable touch of spice to balance the flavors in the smoothie.

Spinach: Packed in vitamins, minerals, and antioxidants, yet hardly detectable until blended into the smoothie.

Place your banana and mixed berries in a blender to begin making your Berry Spinach Protein Smoothie.Add the Greek yogurt, plain, next.then your preferred protein powder.flaxseed meal as well.Put down your leafy greens after that.Add some ginger and cinnamon on top.Blend in ice and a small amount of water until smooth.Evenly pour into glasses, present, and savor!

19.   CRANBERRY   CLEANSE SMOOTHIE

The Cranberry Detox Smoothie is an easy and tasty smoothie recipe that uses anti-inflammatory vitamins and minerals to help cleanse the body.

This Cranberry Detox Smoothie is a terrific smoothie recipe to try if you're trying to get back on track with a healthy diet. Made with just a few nutritious ingredients, this smoothie recipe is a terrific last-minute breakfast choice. This is the time of year when fresh cranberries may be found in stores for a great price. Because cranberries are high in vitamins, fiber, and other minerals, this smoothie is ideal for the body's detoxification and nourishment.

Components

- Frozen fresh cranberries, one cup
- One apple, cored and peeled
- Half a cup almond milk (or any other type of milk)
- Half a cup water and half a teaspoon of ground cinnamon
- Half a teaspoon of turmeric powder

Directions

In a large blender, add all the ingredients and process until smooth.

If preferred, garnish with cranberries and ground cinnamon.

20. ALOE VERA DIGESTIVE DETOX

Aloe vera has several benefits for the digestive system, including bowel movement, less bloating, relief from constipation, and prevention of diarrhea. These benefits are crucial for detoxifying and preventing the accumulation of toxins. While aloe vera gel is collected straight from the leaves of the plant, aloe juice is typically made from the entire leaf and may contain more water. Fresh aloe vera gel is the best choice for smoothies since it has a creamier texture and a higher vitamin concentration.

Basic Recipe for Aloe Vera Smoothie

- Two teaspoons of aloe juice or a quarter cup of fresh aloe vera gel
- One cup of coconut milk or water
- One cup of frozen berry mixture (strawberries, raspberries, and blueberries).
- One little banana
- One tablespoon of agave nectar or honey(optional).

Blend to desired texture and enjoy!

21. LEMON-GINGER ZEST SMOOTHIE

The potent qualities of fresh lemon, ginger, yogurt, and honey are combined in this lemon ginger smoothie to create a nutritious breakfast that can combat anything winter throws at you, including the flu and dry skin!

To be healthy, a smoothie doesn't have to be thick and runny or loaded with strange powders and additives. Four whole foods make this one light, refreshing, and supercharged. Although none of these nutrients is a miracle cure, they are all potent parts of a balanced diet, and the medical establishment is always researching their fabled health advantages.

INGREDIENTS

YOGURT: T-cells, which defend the body against infections, depend on amino acids in protein for proper activity. Probiotics, or good bacteria, are found in yogurt and can strengthen the immune system and maintain gastrointestinal health. Check the label for the terms "live active cultures" or "probiotics."

Extra points for adding vitamin D to your yogurt to strengthen your immune system.

LEMON: Packed with antioxidants and vitamin C, lemons are a powerful nutrient. Since you'll be using the zest, it would be wise to pick an organic lemon.

GINGER: high in antioxidants and vitamin C as well. It aids with digestion, particularly when consumed empty-handed. Its potential antiviral and antibacterial qualities are being researched. Utilize fresh ginger for maximum benefits.

HONEY: an antibacterial, anti-inflammatory, and antioxidant substance. Honey is frequently taken orally to relieve coughs. The most antioxidant-rich honey is raw honey, so seek it out.

RECIPES AND INSTRUCTIONS

Rinse your lemon well after washing it in sudsy water.

Using a vegetable peeler, remove the zest in strips (only the yellow part, leave the bitter white pith behind). Best used with a serrated peeler.

Cut a knob of ginger into pieces after peeling it. Note: Peeling is optional; it's simply my choice.

In a blender, add rind, ginger, yogurt, honey, lemon juice, and a few ice cubes.

Mix until homogeneous.

22. ALGAE BLUE-GREEN ELIXIR

In addition to being the planet's richest source of chlorophyll, Blue-Green Algae Elixir contains a complete protein. It improves mood and helps the brain operate.Elixir of the Lake's blue-green algae offers special and advantageous nutrients, such as a high protein content, beta-carotenes, B vitamins, chlorophyll, trace minerals, omega-3s, and other useful elements. Encourage your body to rid itself of pollutants naturally to maintain maximum health. Pure Lake Elixir from HealthForce Nutritionals uses nutrient-dense, health-promoting blue green algae to support healthy body cleansing.

Components

- one-half cup almond milk

- One frozen, ripe banana
- One cup of chunks of frozen pineapple
- a half-cup of cucumber slices
- A single tsp of peanut butter
- Two tsp powdered blue-green algae
- Two dates with medjool pits removed

Directions

Put all ingredients in a high-speed blender and blend. Blend until smooth, about 40–45 seconds. To get the right consistency, add more almond milk. Add fresh blackberries on top. Serve right away. Have fun!

23.   POMEGRANATE   PASSION SMOOTHIE

Components

- Two ounces of newly squeezed POM Wonderful (pomegranate juice) Whole Juice of Pomegranates
- Six-ounce nonfat yogurt
- Fresh strawberries in a cup
- Scoop of ice

PREPARATION

1. If needed, make fresh pomegranate juice. In a blender, combine all ingredients and process until desired consistency is reached.

Present and savor!

OR

2. Use a citrus peeler or juicer to juice two to three large POM Wonderful Pomegranates in half to make fresh pomegranate juice. Pour the mixture through a sieve or strainer lined with cheesecloth. Reserve the juice.

24. Pineapple-Mint Slim Down

Components:

1½ to 1 cup water, unsweetened, carrageenan-free almond milk, or canned coconut milk

1/2 a lemon, 1/2 an avocado, or 1/3 cup of full-fat coconut milk from a can

One mound Flavorless Collagen Protein by Dr. Kellyann

One cup of unsweetened pineapple pieces, either fresh, frozen, or canned

six or seven new mint leaves

Grated and peeled ½-inch piece of fresh ginger (optional)

One cup or two handfuls of baby spinach, diced, and monk fruit sweetener or Stevia to taste

Smoothie over ice, add to blender, or combine with ice

Instructions:

Blend together the water, ice (if used), avocado, collagen powder, pineapple, mint, ginger, spinach, and lemon juice (if using) in a blender. Blend till creamy and smooth. To get the right consistency, add more liquid of your choice if the smoothie is too thick.

Take note:

Use ⅓ cup of almond or coconut milk, vanilla protein powder, and canned coconut milk if you like your smoothies creamy.

25. MATCHA GREEN TEA ZEN

Check out these smoothie recipes with matcha green tea powder! These are scrumptious and nutritious ways to boost your energy and vegetable intake!

Matcha will improve your mood, raise your energy level, and speed up your metabolism!

Ingredients for Strawberry Banana Matcha Green Tea Powder Smoothie

- Two cups of frozen strawberries, thawed
- One banana
- One Kiwi, peeled
- Two scoops of protein powder with vanilla flavor
- Half a cup of vanilla almond milk without sugar or half a cup of plain low-fat yogurt
- Two tsp pure virgin olive oil
- Two teaspoons of fine culinary matcha

Blend until they are smooth.

One of our favorite breakfast smoothies is this matcha green tea smoothie!

Ingredients for the recipe for Cacao Matcha Green Tea Powder Smoothie

- 1.5 cups of almond milk without sugar
- One spoonful of powdered cacao
- Half a spoonful of matcha Zen Green tea
- Two tsp powdered maca

Note: You can add a half of a spoonful of maple syrup to the smoothie if you want it to have a little sweetness to counterbalance the bitter cacao. I occasionally add a handful of spinach to my smoothie for an added iron boost, but you don't have to.

YOUTHFUL SKIN MATCHA GREEN TEA POWDER

Components:

- One cup of unflavored almond milk
- One cup of packed baby kale
- Half an avocado, peeled and pittedview_6084

* 1 pitted nectarine
* One cup of berries
* One spoonful of natural almond butter, unsalted
* Two teaspoons of matcha green tea powder (Zen Green Tea)

Blend all ingredients in a blender until they are smooth.

MATCHA GREEN TEA POWDER SMOOTHIE BLUEBERRY COCONUT

Components:

* Coconut aqueous
* One cup frozen blueberries,
* one banana,
* Half cup of fresh spinach,
* and ½ teaspoon of Zen matcha powderHalf.

SMOOTHIE HONEY MATCHA Green Tea Powder

You'll require:

- A tsp of matcha Zen Green Tea
- a pair of teaspoons heated water
- One milk cup.
- Overripe banana
- One-third teaspoon honey
- Four ice cubes

Getting ready:

The matcha powder should first be dissolved in hot water. Next, put all the ingredients in the blender and process them until a smooth consistency is achieved.

SMOOTHIE BANANA MATCHA GREEN TEA POWDER

You'll require:

- One frozen banana that has been peeled and ideally overripe
- A half-cup of milk.

- Matcha half a teaspoon of Zen Green Tea
- You can also taste and add sweeteners and vanilla extract if you'd like.

Getting ready:

In a blender, combine all of the ingredients listed above and process until smooth. If required, stir as well.

MATCHA FRUIT SMOOTHIE POWDER GREEN TEA

You'll require:

- A quarter of a cup of berries, either black, blue, or raspberry-flavored
- A half-cup yogurt
- A half-cup of cubes
- A tsp of matcha Zen Green Tea

Getting ready:

Using an electric blender, combine the ingredients; transfer the mixture into a tall class. It is best to consume it right away after cooking.

Depending on your tastes, you can add kiwis, bananas, mangos, and flavors like ginger or mint.

SMOOTHIE WITH TRADITIONAL MATCHA GREEN TEA POWDER

You'll require:

- A half-cup yogurt
- Two teaspoons sugar or honey
- A half-cup of cubes
- A tsp of matcha Zen Green Tea

Getting ready:

Simply combine all the ingredients in the blender and blend until well combined. That's it, too! Savor your tasty, easy-to-make matcha smoothie.

MATCHA GREEN TEA POWDER CHOCOLATE SMOOTHIE

Components:

Two teaspoons of cocoa powder, oats, ½ cup of banana, one almond milk, one cup of Zen green tea matcha green tea, A splash of sea salt, a pinch of vanilla extract, and ice are optional.

Mix until homogeneous.

Matcha Green Tea Powder with Ginger Infusion Smoothie

Components:

Green Tea Zen Matcha Green Tea, a teaspoon of freshly grated or chopped ginger, two tablespoons of orange juice, a cup of freshly squeezed lime juice, or a spoonful of honey, as needed for sweetness

Blend until smooth with ice.

26. CREAMY BUTTERNUT SQUASH

The butternut squash smoothie is creamy and luscious, with overtones of cinnamon and cardamom that are nicely balanced by strawberries and ginger for a wonderful seasonal drink.

Personally, I prefer smoothies that are bright and refreshing rather than overly indulgent, as if you were drinking a milkshake.

INGREDIENTS

- frozen butternut squash (cooked or roasted earlier)
- strawberries that have been frozen
- almond milk (or other preferred milk) frozen riced cauliflower
- If desired, use pumpkin seed butter, macadamia nut butter, or cashew butter for the almond butter.
- Chia and flax seeds
- dates from the Medjool tree
- Vanilla extract fresh ginger cinnamon cardamom (optional) collagen peptides or protein powder of choice

Although I have smoothies for breakfast virtually every day, I'm finally back with another recipe, this time for a great seasonal smoothie that I think you'll enjoy.

If you think putting butternut squash in a smoothie is strange, this recipe will hopefully prove you wrong.

Using frozen squash, such as butternut squash, is a terrific way to thicken up smoothies and give them a creamy texture. Not to mention the additional health benefits, such as fiber, that they provide!

There are plenty of pumpkin smoothies out there (including my own pumpkin banana smoothie), but most are too spiced and taste like you're drinking pumpkin pie.

This butternut squash smoothie is a touch out of the ordinary. While it has some fall spices, it also contains frozen strawberries and fresh ginger to offset the rich aromas with some refreshing and bright ingredients.

HOW SHOULD BUTTERNUT SQUASH BE FROZEN FOR SMOOTHIES?

There are two ways to freeze the butternut squash for this smoothie.

The simplest option is to purchase cooked frozen butternut squash from the freezer aisle. If your grocer sells it, it's ideal for quick smoothies. Nuzest is my go-to for plant-based protein powders. I really appreciate Paleo Valley's bone broth protein powder for animal protein.

DATES - In this recipe, I normally use 1 medjool date. Use 2 or 3 if you prefer things sweeter. Maple syrup or honey can also be used in place of the sugar.

FROZEN CAULIFLOWER - If you're curious about this ingredient, don't worry, you won't taste any cauliflower at all. I frequently use riced cauliflower in porridge (like this apple cinnamon oatmeal, which is presently on repeat) and smoothies. It's a terrific method to bulk up a meal while also sneaking in some nutrition. Most people put spinach in their smoothies, but cauliflower is the way to go. It also doesn't change the color of whatever you're preparing, which is perfect for fooling small palates.

GINGER - Fresh is ideal, but ground ginger spice can be substituted if you don't have any on hand. The amounts are listed on the recipe card below.

Simply add all ingredients in a high-powered blender and blend until smooth. Pour into a glass or bowl, top with anything you want, and enjoy!

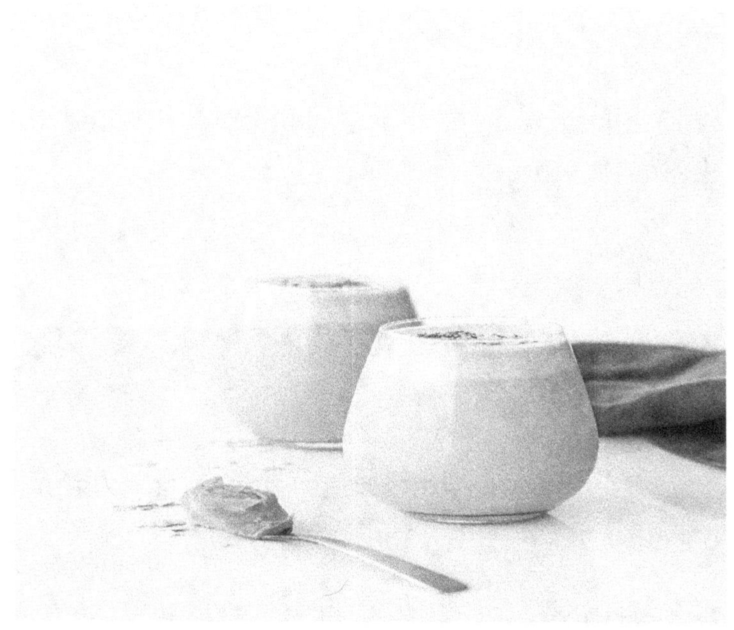

27. STRAWBERRY FLAXSEED INFUSION SMOOTHIE

Strawberry FlaxSeed Smoothie is a quick breakfast made with strawberries, banana, honey, spinach, and nutty flax seeds; only 8 ingredients total! Gluten-free and healthy.

INSTRUCTIONS

Add all ingredients in a blender and blend till desired texture.

28. CUCUMBER-CELERY COOL DOWN

This is one of your go-to things in summer because of its high liquid contents.

Ingredients

2 ozs12 Spinach, 2 cucumber stalks, 14 ounces celery, 1 bunch pineapple flesh, 1 teaspoon Cress, 1 teaspoon LimeMatcha green tea powder, 2 tbsp almonds.

Steps for Preparation

1. Wash and shake dry the spinach. Clean, wash, and chop half a cucumber and celery. Make tiny slices of pineapple flesh. Remove the cress from the bed. Cut the lime in half and squeeze out the juice.
2. In a stand mixer, combine 14 ounces of water, spinach, cucumber, celery, pineapple, lime juice, matcha tea powder, almonds, and cress.

Serve the smoothie in four glasses.

29. MORINGA MAGIC

You get out of bed prepared to face the world and face a new day. However, are you aware of what could make you feel even better and work more effectively throughout the day? Naturally, a strawberry-mango smoothie for spring! To make this smoothie, just follow these easy five steps before starting your day.

Recipe for a Magic Moringa Smoothie:

1) Fill a blender with 1 cup coconut milk, 1.5 bananas, pineapple, 1 mango, and 10 strawberries. These fruits will add a ton of vitamins and antioxidants to your smoothie.

2) Add a tablespoon of chia seeds. Chia seeds are rich in omega-3 fatty acids and fiber. To optimize your body's absorption of chia seeds' nutrients, make sure to purchase them whole and ground them right before using. While a coffee grinder works well in many situations, you can also use a blender to combine smoothie ingredients.

3) Add one scoop of your preferred whey protein flavor to stay full. My favorite flavor in this smoothie is vanilla!

4) Of course, incorporate the powdered moringa.

5) Blend and savor!

30. ALMOND JOY DELIGHT

For breakfast, a candy bar? That'd be insane. Savor the delight of almonds combined with coconut and chocolate syrup to create a sweet yet filling smoothie that can be consumed as a morning meal.

INGREDIENTS

- Sweetened Vanilla Almond Milk, 8 fl. oz.,
- 5.25 ounces of vanilla Greek yogurt
- Four ounces of chocolate syrup
- One cup of sweetened, flakes coconut Sliced Almonds, 1 oz.
- Chia seeds, 1 tablespoon

Blend Components

Set aside a little portion of almonds and coconut flakes for decorating. Put everything in the blender, excluding the chocolate sauce. Blend until smooth, about 2 minutes on high.Put the Ice in

After adding two cups of ice, mix for a further thirty to sixty seconds. Close and raise a glass!

Drizzle two glasses, bottom and sides, with half of the chocolate sauce. Spoon smoothie into each glass. Top with shaved almonds and coconut flakes, then drizzle with remaining chocolate sauce.